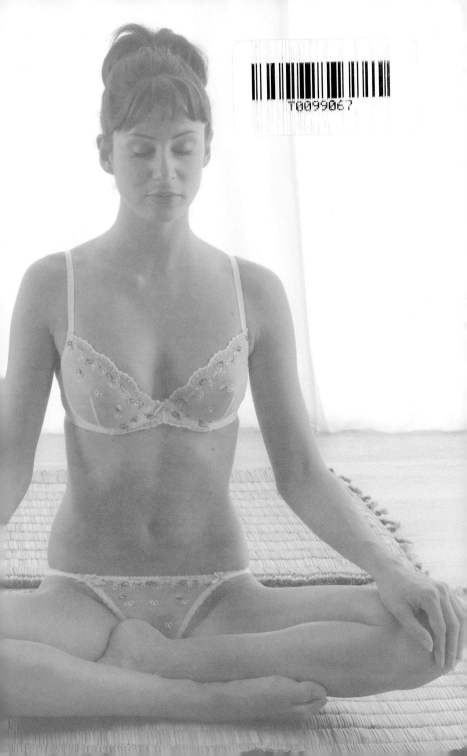

50 natural ways to
feel sexy

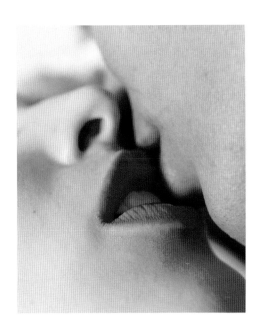

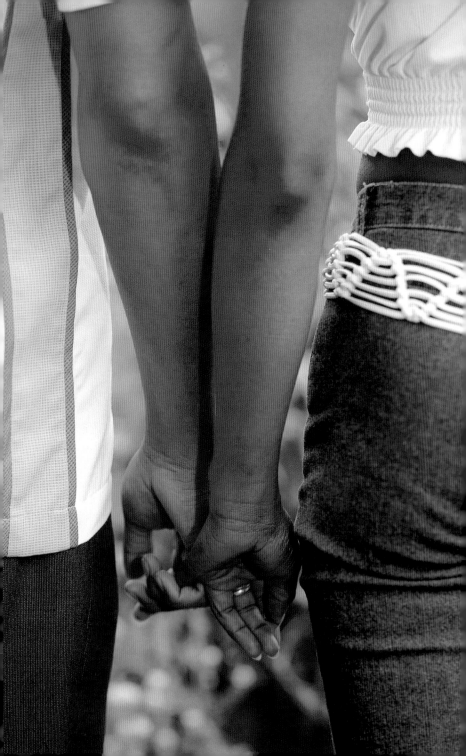

50 natural ways to
feel sexy

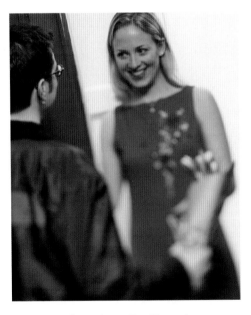

Jessica Dolland

LORENZ BOOKS

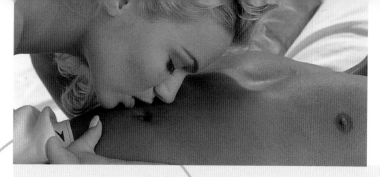

contents

INTRODUCTION 6

INCREASING SEXUAL DESIRE 10
FEELING GOOD

1) the game of seduction 12
2) date your partner 13
3) time together 14
4) re-vamp your image 15
5) stress busting exercise 16
6) tension-relieving stretches 17
7) sexercises 18
8) mind-clearing meditation 19
9) boost your confidence 20
10) sleep strategies 21

VITALITY BOOSTERS

11) supple sensuality 22
12) dynamic breath 23
13) herbs to give you a lift 24
14) help from homeopathy 25
15) flower essences for fun 26
16) crystal energy focus 27
17) reflexology energizer 28
18) high-energy eating 29

feel sexy

MOOD FOODS

19) erotic feasts   30

20) exotics and curiosities   31

21) seductive salads   32

22) asparagus to share   33

23) luxurious seafood   34

24) turning up the heat   35

25) nuts and honey   36

26) irresistible chocolate   37

27) chocolate-dipped fruit   38

28) fruity passion   39

29) popping corks   40

SEDUCTIVE BEAUTY TREATMENTS

30) aromatherapy bath oils   41

31) smooth silky skin   42

32) scented bubbles   43

33) delicious dusting powder   44

34) shimmering tresses   45

35) mint foot treatments   46

AROUSING THE SENSES

36) colour magic   47

37) setting the scene   48

38) create a love nest   49

39) romantic lighting   50

40) scents for seduction   51

41) sexy essential oils   52

SENSUAL PLEASURES

42) pillow talk   53

43) loving face massage   54

44) sensual touch   55

45) kissing asides   56

46) ice fire   57

47) sexplorations   58

48) playing games   59

49) erotica   60

50) sharing fantasies   61

INDEX   62

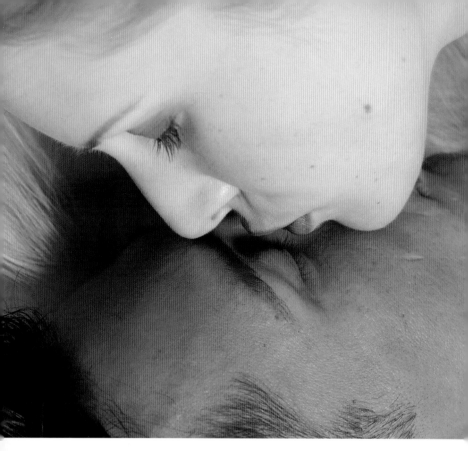

introduction

We are sexual beings, and sexiness is thoroughly enmeshed with every aspect of our lives. Feeling sexy is all about feeling good about yourself, and this book suggests some simple ways to help you do that, with tips on using a range of complementary therapies and natural remedies.

You may feel that your general level of health is good, but a little extra effort can really supercharge your body. Stepping up the amount of exercise you do, and re-jigging your diet to include more high-energy

foods, will quickly boost your metabolism, improving your cardio-vascular and respiratory health and balancing your hormones. Feeling fit and looking great is a real tonic for self-esteem, lifting the spirits and increasing zest for life.

When you're stressed, or depressed or tired, all kinds of pleasure can go out of the window. But a lack of sexual desire could also be induced by drugs. If you smoke, you're probably already familiar with all the good reasons why you need to give it up: the

◄ *Introducing seductive techniques, and playful, loving behaviour can kick start a sluggish sex life in a long-term relationship.*

effect on your sex life is just one of them. Smoking causes constriction of the blood vessels, and the consequent lowering of blood flow to the pelvic region leads to a decrease of sexual arousal in both men and women. Studies have found that in men between the ages of thirty and fifty, smoking increases the risk of impotence by fifty per cent.

Alcohol can also be a problem. Most drinkers would agree that a glass or two puts them in the mood for sex: they feel relaxed and shed any inhibitions. But heavy drinking has the opposite effect. Antidepressants, oral contraceptives and caffeine in coffee and fizzy drinks can also diminish your sex drive.

sex and sensuality

We talk about sexiness as a feeling, but rather than relaxing into that feeling we spend a great deal of time thinking about it instead. These days we are surrounded by images of sex: in films, on television, in magazines. Raunchy photographs and innuendo-laced slogans glare down from advertising hoardings, selling everything from cars to coffee. This kind of thing is part of the landscape and most people don't find it much of a thrill.

Good sex is about much more than the mechanics of coupling. It's about communication, confidence, a level of sensitivity and a sense of humour. Most of all it's about sensuality: the

engaging of all the senses to enable you to enjoy your own body and share that total enjoyment with your partner. There are plenty of ways to introduce more sensuality to your sex life. By concentrating on all five senses, you can find ways to make them all tingle with pleasure.

Be aware of the pressure of your touch when caressing your lover, from the gentlest brush of the fingertips to firmer strokes. Experience the feeling of different textures on your skin, such as the cool, slippery feel of silk or the

▼ *Take long hot baths with your partner, and unwind together after a stressful day.*

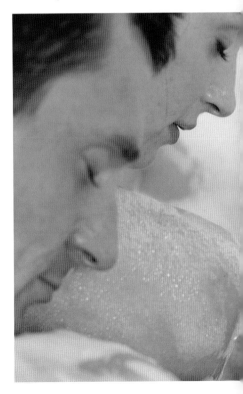

softness of velvet; play around with feathers, rubber, a soft brush.

Choose music to go with your mood. Mellow jazz or gentle classical music could help you unwind and relax. Brazilian or Cuban music is very sensual and can strongly influence the way you move together. Stimulate your sense of sight with atmospheric lighting such as candles or flickering firelight, creating an effect that flatters and pleases both of you. Explore all the contours of your bodies with your eyes, and watch your shadows moving on the wall.

The sense of smell has a powerful influence on your mood and emotions, and is especially important in the intimacy of lovemaking. The best smell is the smell of sex – that musky, heavy, natural perfume that attracts us to one another. But you can also rub musk or vanilla scented oil into your skin, perfume your hair, burn incense or light scented candles with sensuous aromas such as jasmine or sandalwood.

You'll be particularly sensitive to the taste of your bodies, but you might also enjoy some delicious morsels to tempt each other. Choose contrasting flavours and sensations: the satin smoothness of melting chocolate, the juicy tang of ripe mangoes, the salty slipperiness of oysters, the softness of cream, the sweet cold of ice cream.

This kind of delight in sensual pleasure isn't something to confine to sexual experience. A greater general sensual awareness can heighten your enjoyment of every daily activity, restoring your spirits and making you feel truly alive.

▾ Sensual massage is an obvious start to sex, and can also be a good way to unwind.

▸ Make your evening routine something special with candlelight and wine.

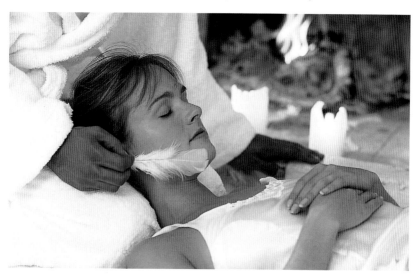

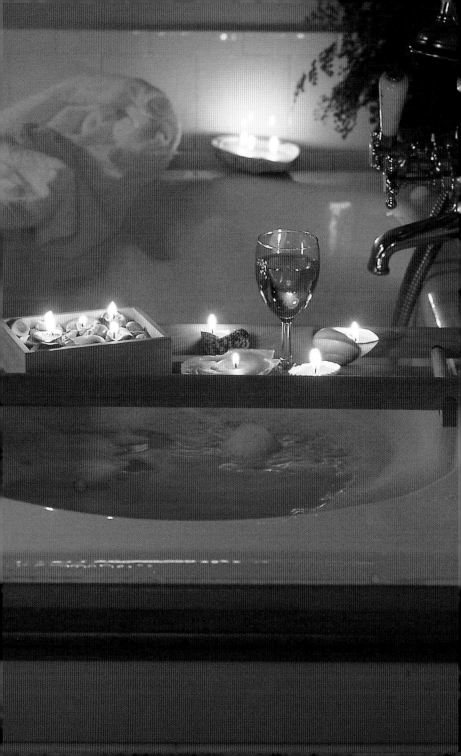

increasing
sexual desire

The quest for sure-fire aphrodisiacs is as old as humanity. Sexual desire is such a slippery commodity, and so important to our happiness, that every culture on earth seems to have developed its own repertoire of arousing foods, drinks and other remedies. Without making any claims for their efficacy, this book includes some of the most famous of these magic bullets – from oysters to chillies to the scent of jasmine. They might just work for you, and even if they don't they're fun to try.

The book also outlines a range of tried-and-tested natural therapies and remedies to tackle specific problems such as tiredness and stress, together with lots of delicious ideas to stimulate all your senses, from lighting your bedroom to scenting your bath. And finally, when you've made it to bed, there are some light-hearted suggestions for you and your lover to play around with. Sex is, after all, meant to be fun.

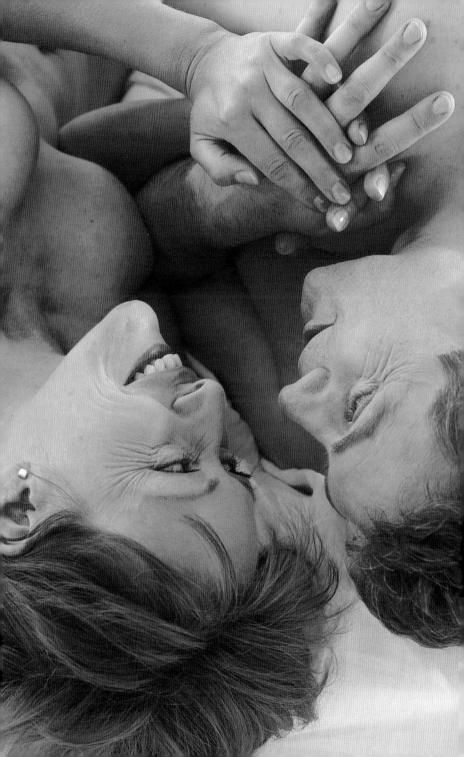

1

the game of seduction

It's often said that sex is ten per cent physical and ninety per cent emotional – the true foundations of sensuality, sexual enjoyment and fulfilment lie in the brain.

Unlike most animals, humans have sex for recreation, comfort and love, as well as for procreation. Preparation, anticipation and relaxation all start in the head: we need to be in the mood for sex, and this is controlled by the brain, the erotic epicentre of the body.

Dating, romancing, courting and flirting may seem a little old-fashioned to some people, but everyone is susceptible. Romance doesn't have to be flowers, toys and soppy letters. Small, thoughtful gestures usually have a far greater impact than large, lavish ones.

In the early stages of a relationship you can think of little else but each other and all your senses are alive with anticipation. The sky seems bluer, flowers smell sweeter and jokes seem funnier. Great memories are made during this period of getting to know one another, and can be evoked for ever after by a particular smell or a line of music. It is a sad fact that the better you get to know someone the more complacent you become about romance, but in a longstanding relationship it can still be disarming and delightful, and it is worth making the effort to revive it.

▾ *In the early stages of a relationship your focus on each other is strong and intense.*

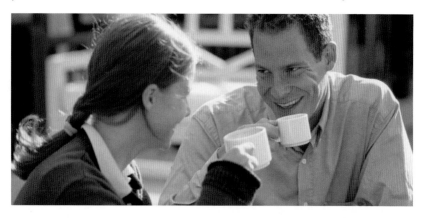

date your partner

However long you've been in a relationship, **regular dating** keeps you feeling important to each other – remember how **excited** you felt the **first time** you went out together?

3

time together

However busy your lives, it's important to make time when your lives are not just running along parallel tracks. Take a walk with no fixed destination. Spend time together without pressure.

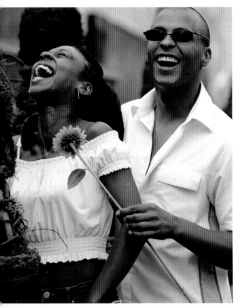

▲ Give your relationship the space it needs to be spontaneous and fun.

The ancient eastern philosophy of Tantra embraces sexuality as a means of reaching spiritual enlightenment, and cultivates the art of sex as a skilled spiritual practice. It sees sex as an expression of union, not just between you and your partner but with the whole of existence.

The pressures of modern life can leave you feeling isolated and unable to relate to each other or to experience each moment fully. Taking time out to renew your relationship with nature can help you feel that you are both part of the same whole and resolve that sense of separation.

at one with nature

Submerge yourselves in nature and renew your sense of wonder by making a serious commitment to break away from the daily responsibilities of work and home, and rediscover the magic of the natural world.

Lie on a beach on a warm moonlit night to gaze at the stars and listen to the roar of the waves. Walk through a forest and explore the myriad lives that coexist within it, or stroll across a soft carpet of meadow grass searching for wild flowers and becoming aware of the jubilant birdsong above you. Sit by a river and watch insects dance and buzz above the water. Feel yourselves to be part of the splendour of nature and carry this awareness into your love-making.

4 re-vamp your image

When you catch sight of yourself in a mirror you feel great if it gives you a buzz. If you've stopped noticing, it's time to splash out and make some changes – one change can lead to another.

It's said that beauty comes from within – and it does – but it can work the other way too. Knowing you look lovely puts a spring in your step, and its effect on your whole approach to life could surprise you.

Advertisers promise "a whole new you" with every new beauty product: the fashion and beauty industries are founded on our insecurities about our appearance, and both men and women are susceptible. A makeover won't transform your life, but it can be a great morale-boost, helping you see yourself as the sexy person you are.

Most people wear their hair the same way for years without changing it. A change of style can be a real tonic. You'll get noticed and complimented – with luck by your partner, but certainly by everyone else. Consider changing the colour too. It's amazing what a difference even the softest tint can make to your hair, your face and your overall image.

When you shop for clothes, dare to try on colours and styles you wouldn't normally choose. And buying sexy underwear might seem like a cliché, but it works.

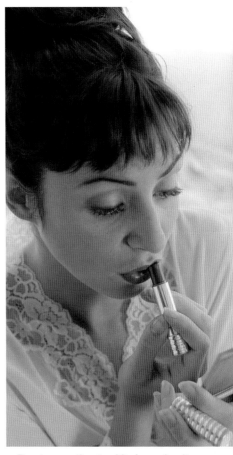

▲ Devote some time to a bit of preening, it will boost your self-esteem amazingly.

5 stress-busting exercise

Great sex goes with good health, and an important aspect of keeping well is keeping fit. Regular exercise will not only keep your body in shape but will reduce stress and make you happier.

Jogging, swimming, cycling and walking are all excellent aerobic sports. The most important thing is to choose a form of exercise that you enjoy so that it's no problem finding time for regular sessions – there's no point in joining a gym if you stop going after a few weeks. Don't overdo things, but start gently and gradually build up your stamina, strength and suppleness. Try to make some exercise a part of your daily routine, even if it's just a brisk walk on your way to work.

Exercise is just as important when you're young as when you are older, and you will benefit by keeping your heart and lungs strong and your muscles toned. Aerobic exercise burns fat, boosts the immune system, aids flexibility and improves sleep, making you feel healthier, livelier and sexier.

freeing the mind

As well as toning your body, exercise is good for your mind. It's a great stress-reliever, distracting you from nagging anxieties and, by releasing tension in your body, helping to free up your mind too. Vigorous activity causes a rise in the level of endorphins in the blood and these substances, the body's natural painkillers, are thought to be connected with feelings of euphoria and the release of sex hormones. (Endorphins are also produced during sex.) The sense of achievement you get after exercise will raise your self-esteem, you'll feel proud of your fitter body – and happy to show it off.

◄ Exercising together is a great way to create a bond while improving fitness.

6 tension-relieving stretches

This simple sequence of stretching exercises helps to release tension in the spine and tones all the organs in the pelvic basin, as well as improving blood flow to and from the area.

1 For twisting sit-ups, lie on your back with your legs bent, feet apart, and hands behind your head. Breathe in, then, as you exhale, raise your head and one shoulder, at the same time raising your leg so that opposite elbow and knee approach each other. Lower the shoulder and knee, then repeat on the other side.

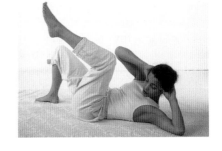

2 Sitting with your legs straight out in front of you, bend one leg and place the foot on the outside of the other leg. Reach around the bent leg with the opposite arm to hold the straight leg and twist your upper body. Relax and repeat on the other side.

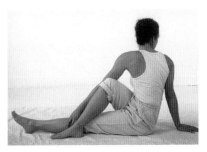

3 Bend both legs and bring the soles of the feet together. Clasp the feet with your hands and try to pull them a little closer to your body. Let the knees drop towards the floor. Hold the stretch, relax and repeat.

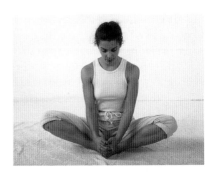

7 sexercises

Like any other muscles, the pelvic floor muscles need to be kept toned. Apart from enhancing your sex life, a strong pelvic floor avoids problems with bladder and bowel control in later life.

The pubococcygeus (PC) muscle resembles a hammock slung between the legs, and is the one that contracts at a rate of just under once a second during orgasm. It tends to become flabbier with age, and other factors – childbirth, weight gain or a chronic cough – can weaken it further.

for her

Exercises designed to strengthen the pelvic muscles and tighten the vagina were practised by women in ancient China and India. Kegel exercises, which are now widely used, were devised by Dr Arnold Kegel in 1948 as a means of reducing incontinence after childbirth, but they can also help intensify and prolong orgasms.

You first need to locate and isolate the correct muscle, and the easiest way to do this is to stop and start the flow while urinating (although you should not do Kegel exercises during urination). Exercise by tightening and relaxing the muscle twenty times in a session and build up to sixty or more. Then prolong each squeeze to five seconds. You can do them anywhere: on a train, in the office, or in bed.

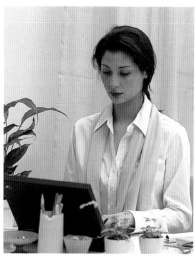

▲ Pelvic floor exercises are totally discreet, can be done almost anywhere.

for him

Kegel exercises are also suitable for men. An additional exercise is to place a small damp towel on your erect penis and practise moving it up and down. Strong pelvic floor muscles give you greater control over the timing of your orgasm, and a recent study of older men has shown that pelvic floor exercises can help to restore erectile function.

8

mind-clearing meditation

Just one session of meditation can leave you feeling refreshed and happier, and long-term practice can transform your life. Make it a daily habit. You can practise alone or with your partner.

Meditation is a way of focusing the mind and stilling the mental chatter that distracts us from concentrated attention. Even while we're enjoying something, we're only half there, with part of our mind wandering along other tracks. Meditating helps us to live in the moment.

alpha waves

Each time you meditate, your heart slows, your blood pressure drops and your brain starts to produce alpha waves. You may have experienced the alpha state by chance when you were very relaxed. When you slip into it you feel a sense of deep contentment. Niggling worries vanish. Meditation is a simple technique for finding that calm space whenever you need it.

learning to meditate

It's easiest to get into the meditation habit if you do it at the same time and place every day. It doesn't have to take long: set a timer for ten minutes once a day. The simplest way to start is to

count your breaths. Sit comfortably with your back straight and let your breathing slow down, then count the length of each breath just before you take a new one. Count up to ten, then start again. Keep your attention on your breathing. Note how the air feels as it enters and leaves your body. As thoughts enter your mind, let them drift away. Before long it becomes easier to bring your focus back after each detour. You stop fidgeting and begin to feel a sense of peace.

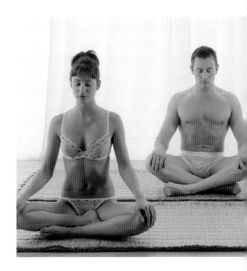

▸ *Try a joint meditation session as a prelude to making love.*

9 boost your confidence

Don't wait to hear compliments from others: just tell yourself you're great. Emphasize all your positive attributes and you'll see what an attractive and irresistible person you really are.

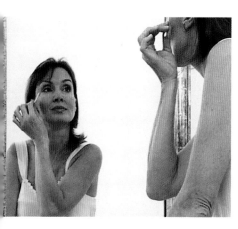

◄ Build your affirmations into your usual morning or evening routines.

Lack of confidence can dull your sexual energy and enjoyment just as it limits your potential in other aspects of life. Feeling really good about yourself has the opposite effect. If you are a severe self-critic you already know how influential your own voice is, because you believe it. You can use its power to emphasize your positive aspects instead. Making affirmations during meditation is a deceptively simple but effective device that can change the way you think about yourself and the way you act.

The technique requires you to say out loud, positive statements about yourself as you wish to be. Be aware of any negative statements you habitually make, such as "I find it hard to talk to people," or "I am too fat". You are reinforcing these self-limiting beliefs each time they slip into your conversation, but you can use affirmations to change such beliefs. The affirmations should be in the present tense and should be positively phrased.

- I like my... [eyes/hair/legs...]
- I am proud of my... [intelligence/sense of humour/achievement]
- My friendship is valuable to... [name of person]
- I am lovable and can give love.

Keeping the statements short will give them more impact. You don't have to believe them at first, but if you repeat them often enough, they start to make a difference. Belief will come and your feeling of self-worth will grow.

10 sleep strategies

Feeling too tired to make love at the end of the day is a common problem. Stress and overwork can cause a loss of libido and can also result in insomnia, creating a vicious cycle of tiredness.

▸ *Making sure you both get enough sleep will improve your energy levels in all areas.*

To break the stress cycle, learning to relax needs to be built into a daily pattern that also makes time for healthy meals and some regular exercise. It may be that only one of you is having disturbed nights, but relaxing rituals that prepare you for sleep are a pleasure to share.

Make your bedroom as calm and serene as possible, banning the television, computers and work-related clutter to create a peaceful, secure cocoon. Avoid eating late at night, and instead of tea or coffee try a relaxing herbal infusion. Unwind in a warm bath – together if you like – scented with a blend of sedative essential oils such as rose, lavender and ylang ylang. Read a novel or listen to gentle music to take your mind off the concerns of the day before you settle down and try to sleep.

If you do wake during the night, don't just lie there allowing yourself to get tense and panicky. If a heavy workload is causing stress, one way to free your mind at night is to write

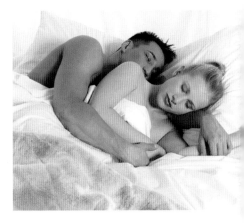

down a list of all the tasks you need to do tomorrow so that you can stop running through them in your head.

post-coital sleep

Of course, sex itself can be an effective aid to falling asleep – particularly for men. If you are a woman who enjoys that precious relaxed time of lying together, having a partner who falls instantly asleep can be exasperating. On the other hand, you could choose to see it as an indication of his total security and trust in you, and just enjoy lying next to him in a warm glow until you drift off to sleep too.

11 supple sensuality

Yoga works to integrate mind, body and spirit. The regular postures of hatha yoga can help you to relax or feel more energetic. For a surge of energy work through dynamic poses such as the Warrior.

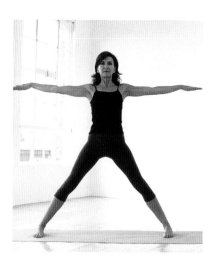

1 Stand with feet together and arms at your side, inhale deeply, and jump or step the feet 1–1.2m/3–4ft apart, and raise the arms to shoulder level. Turn the palms upwards and extend the arms towards the ceiling, keeping the elbows straight and the palms facing one another. Turn the right foot and leg in deeply, about 40 degrees, and the left foot out 90 degrees. At the same time, turn the hips, trunk and shoulders to the left. Both sides of the trunk should be parallel – so bring the right hip forwards, while taking the left hip slightly back, to keep them even.

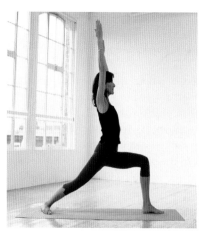

2 Exhale and bend the left leg to form a 90-degree angle. Extend the trunk upwards, as if it were being lifted out of the hips. Move the shoulder blades into the body to open the chest. Extend the chin towards the ceiling and look up. Maintain the full extension on the back leg and keep the hips, shoulders and trunk rotating to the left. Hold for 20–30 seconds, inhale, come up and lower the arms. Repeat on the other side, coming back to the original position, facing forwards with feet together and arms by the side .

12 dynamic breath

Breathing exercises, or pranayama, are an essential aspect of yoga. The breath is considered to carry prana, the life force, around the body to revitalize the entire being.

Our breathing patterns reflect our emotional and mental state. When we are nervous or strained, our breathing tends to be shallow and fast. Taking control of this, and slowing down the breathing calms the nervous system and dissolves stress. Be aware of how you are breathing during the day, and when the rate increases, consciously bring it down to a slower speed. Then try either of these two breathing exercises to revitalize your life force.

alternate nostril breathing

1 Sitting erect, place your right hand against your face. Your eyes may be closed, or open and gazing softly ahead. Close your right nostril with your thumb and breathe in through the left nostril.

2 Release the right nostril and close the left. Breathe out slowly, then in again, through your right nostril. Then open the left nostril, close the right and breathe out. Repeat the sequence five times.

▸ *Breathing exercises just need a few moments of quiet.*

bee breath

This is a relaxing technique that relieves insomnia and produces a meditative state. It can also give you a deliciously sexy voice, as it releases tension in the throat.

1 Sit upright with your eyes closed. Take a long breath in, then breathe out slowly through your nose, making a continuous humming noise.

2 Relax and let the sound become deep and rich. Repeat five times, focusing your mind on the sound.

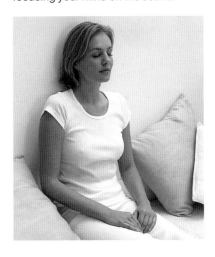

13

herbs to give you a lift

When your libido needs a boost, try a herbal tea. Among medicinal herbs there are several with ancient reputations as aphrodisiacs. They work by invigorating and nourishing the nervous system.

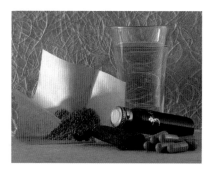

◄ Consulting a herbalist is a good way of making sure you get the right remedy.

korean ginseng (*panax sp.*)

Ginseng – whose name means "wonder of the world" – spurs energy of every kind and increases strength and stamina. By improving the production of adrenal hormones, it helps the body to adapt to stress and fights fatigue. But it should be taken only as a short-term remedy (not more than six weeks).

ENERGIZING TEA

Put 1 tsp dried damiana and 1 tsp dried vervain in a pot and pour on 600ml/1 pint/2 ½ cups boiling water. Steep for 10 minutes then strain and flavour with ginger or honey. Drink two cups a day.

damiana (*turnera diffusa*)

This Central American herb is a traditional remedy for reviving sexual function (it was previously called Turnera aphrodisiaca) as it stimulates the reproductive organs and boosts blood flow. It works as a tonic for both the nervous and hormonal systems,

vervain (*verbena officinalis*)

The Romans considered vervain a magical herb and used it to alleviate depression and nervous exhaustion as well as for its aphrodisiac potency. It has a slightly sedative effect, releasing tension and stress.

wild oats (*avena sativa*)

Oats are an excellent general tonic – they'll give you energy and lift your mood. They're also a good source of vitamin E, iron, zinc, manganese and protein. A traditional breakfast of porridge every morning is a great idea, but there are lots of other delicious ways to eat oats, such as flapjacks and oatcakes.

14 help from homeopathy

Feeling sexually fulfilled is a matter of the mind and emotions as much as physical responses, so if you're having problems with a low sex drive homeopathy might help.

Many people respond positively to homeopathy, which is based on the premise that "like cures like". The remedies are extremely dilute forms of substances that in their normal form would cause the symptoms presented. They're completely safe. Homeopaths treat a person as a whole, not as a list of symptoms, taking into account your character, lifestyle, habits, medical history, and the relationships between all aspects of your life. The prescription is likely to be different in every case, but one of the following remedies might be used for sexual problems.

Agnus castus: for impotence or failure to reach orgasm through fatigue and lack of energy.

Graphites: for men with a positive aversion to sex.

Lycopodium: to help in premature ejaculation or lack of erection.

Sepia: for women who feel irritable, exhausted and indifferent to sex.

Natrum mur: for women who are suffering a loss of libido associated with grief, and who are unable to let go of their emotions.

▾ *The distinctive, tiny homeopathic pills are much easier to take than other medicine.*

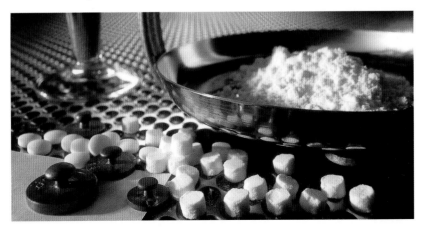

15 flower essences for fun

Sex is bound to be more fun when you're feeling sunny and optimistic. Bach flower remedies harness the natural energy of plants to balance your emotions and cheer you up.

You can swallow a few drops of any or all of the following essences each day to keep your spirits high, and there are other ways in which you and your partner can share their effects. Just add a few drops to a water spray and spritz the bedroom, not forgetting the bed, or add them to a scented bath oil. When you wash clothes and bedlinen, add flower essences to the final rinse.

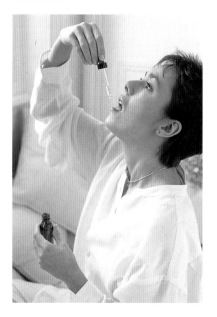

borage
If you're sad, borage cheers you up and makes you feel buoyant and bold.

daffodil
When your ego needs a boost, daffodil essence removes self-doubt and helps you appreciate your own talents, so that life can blossom again.

zinnia
This essence is for people who are taking life too seriously; it restores spontaneity and playfulness and helps you take a detached view — and have a laugh at yourself.

dandelion
Try dandelion when you've too much to do and you're feeling stressed. It will help you relax and give you a feeling of effortless energy.

buttercup
Good for a lack of self-esteem, buttercup warms and nourishes the being with golden light.

◄ *Bach remedies are a gentle and effective way of treating emotional problems.*

16 crystal energy focus

Gemstones have long been recognized as possessing healing properties. Experimenting with different crystals may help you find the one that has a particular resonance for you.

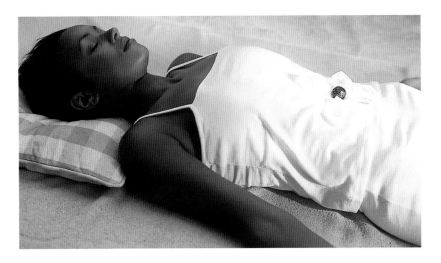

▲ Lying for a few minutes with a red garnet placement will help increase your energy.

The red garnet is the finest energizing stone for the body, especially when it's cut. The facets increase the liveliness of the stone and act like a lens, focusing light with more intensity. Fiery garnet can be placed wherever you feel a lack of energy. It acts as a "starter motor" and very often needs only a short while to do its work.

a balancing placement

After a hard day's work it can sometimes take a long time to "wind down" and feel relaxed enough to enjoy yourself. A simple placement of stones can help you to feel calm and refreshed after a couple of minutes.

Lying down comfortably, place a garnet at the centre of the body and surround it with four clear quartz cyrstals, points facing outwards. The quartz will help increase the garnet's energy and distribute it. Lie in this position for 4–5 minutes, then remove the stones.

17 reflexology energizer

After a reflexology session, most people are deeply relaxed, but soon begin to feel energized and motivated. This is an intimate, caring touch therapy that can awaken your senses.

A foot massage, working on reflexology principles, is a gentle way of establishing touch between you both. For a more vigorous and thorough reflexology session, consult a practitioner.

CAUTION
If you choose to try reflexology on your partner, it is important that he or she is in good health.

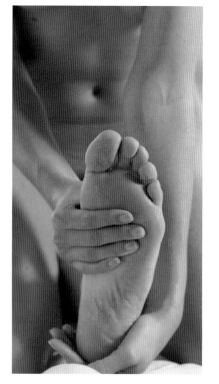

stimulating the body's systems
1 Massage the whole of the feet vigorously to get the circulation going.

2 Applying downward pressure with the tip of the thumb, "thumbwalk" along the instep to stimulate the nervous system in the spinal cord.

3 Work the ball of the foot, corresponding to the chest, to establish regular, deep breathing.

4 Work the pituitary reflex in the centre of the big toe-print: this is the master gland, which controls the other endocrine glands and produces hormones involved in many bodily systems, including sexual functioning.

◀ *You can perform this quick foot massage on yourself or on your partner.*

18 high-energy eating

Boost your sexual energy, as well as your general health, by sticking to a super-nourishing diet rich in fresh, natural foods. Cut down on sugar-rich and salty snacks.

A diet that makes you feel more energetic is based on natural, nutritious, wholesome ingredients, rather than fatty fast foods. To boost your energy levels, snack on fresh and dried fruits that are high in natural sugars, such as pears, kiwi fruit and apricots. Eat plenty of vegetables such as peas, spinach, cabbage and onions.

VITAL VITAMINS AND MINERALS
A well-balanced diet will contain all the vitamins and minerals you need for a healthy libido, including the following:
Vitamin E: protects blood cells and tissues, and may have a direct effect on fertility and sexual function.
Vitamin B3/niacin: acts as a vasodilator, increasing blood flow to the skin.
Vitamin B8/folic acid: assists ovarian function and sperm production.
Zinc: thought to support male prostate function, sperm count and libido.
Selenium: may stimulate sexual energy.
Iodine: supports the thyroid gland, improves desire and capacity.

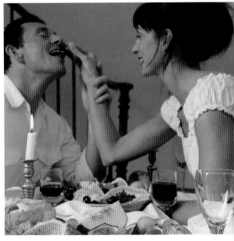

▲ Food can be fun as well as healthy, choose exotic fruit to share together.

Include oily fish, such as salmon and mackerel, poultry and lean red meat such as game and lean beef.

Nuts, brown rice, seeds, pulses and whole grains are packed with energy-giving protein and carbohydrates, they are also rich in valuable minerals and vitamins. Use cold-pressed oils such as olive, grapeseed or sunflower with salads. Don't skip dairy foods but stick to skimmed or semi-skimmed milk and natural low-fat yogurt.

19 erotic feasts

Like great sex, the enjoyment of fantastic food with your partner can be a sublime experience that stimulates all the senses. It makes perfect sense to put the two together.

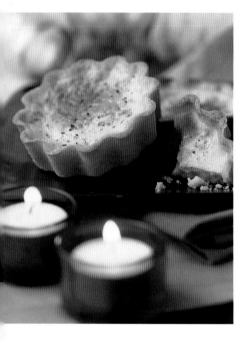

◀ *Small amounts of intensely sweet food will give you a sudden energy burst.*

Choose lovely sensual food, with buttery sauces to glisten alluringly on your lips and titbits that you can proffer to your partner across a candlelit table.

If the prospect of making love wipes away your appetite beforehand, eating after sex can be divine. Sharing food in bed creates a playful, happy atmosphere, and might even give you the energy to start all over again. You can go and raid the fridge together (which you'll have carefully pre-stocked with delicious treats like sushi, mangoes, strawberries and ice cream).

a midnight feast

Prepare a perfect treat – oysters and champagne, say – but hide it from your partner. Have a normal evening with a light meal, then say you're tired and go to bed early. Once your partner's asleep you can sneak out of bed, set the scene with candles and soft music and retrieve the feast from the kitchen. Wake your partner gently and enjoy a night of passion.

Preparing a special meal for your lover is a time-honoured seduction technique. Gazing across the table as you peel a prawn or sink your teeth into a ripe fig can make you both tingle with anticipation. If you're choosing a menu with seduction in mind, keep it light – you don't want to end up full and slumped on the sofa.

20 exotics and curiosities

Is there really such a thing as an aphrodisiac? In every culture, particular delicacies are credited with the ability to drive women mad with passion or give men the stamina to make love all weekend.

Aphrodisiacs are named after the Greek goddess of love, Aphrodite, but the idea is a universal one. Hopeful lovers have enlisted the help of foods and potions of all descriptions, from chocolate to powdered rhino horn.

Rare and exotic foods, particularly, are believed to have this special power. The more outlandish and expensive they are, the better they work – and perhaps there's some truth in this. You may want your lover to realize that you are using an aphrodisiac to seduce him or her, and this could be quite persuasive in itself.

truffles

In one study, women who were shown photographs of men thought they looked sexier when the smell of truffles was wafted past them. To test the effect for yourself, try shavings of fresh black or white truffle scattered over scrambled eggs or fresh pasta.

caviar

The ultimate luxury food: eating it is certainly a sensual experience. It's also rich in zinc, so it could really be good for the male libido.

fugu

The Japanese puffer fish is potentially deadly if not properly prepared, yet it's a costly and much sought-after delicacy. Japanese men take an aphrodisiac potion made by mixing its sperm with hot sake.

snake blood

In parts of Asia it's believed that blood freshly pumped from a dying snake - preferably poisonous – is a potent aphrodisiac. Some bars serve vodka and blood cocktails.

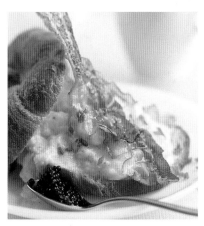

▲ Caviar can be eaten in all kinds of ways and with almost any meal.

21 seductive salads

Plenty of raw food in your diet keeps all the body's systems working at full power, but some salad ingredients just seem to have the edge when it comes to sex.

All fresh, "live" raw vegetables and fruits contain vital enzymes – destroyed by cooking – that enhance digestion and have a great de-toxing effect. Big bowls of exciting salads will keep your skin glowing and your eyes bright, and help you stay lean and lively. For extra sex appeal, try some of these foods, all of which have an overt or more subtle sexual reputation.

When they first reached Europe from South America, tomatoes were known as "love apples". This may have been due to a simple mistranslation, but the link endured, helped by their voluptuous form and colour.

The Aztec name for the avocado means "testicle tree", and their shape, hanging in pairs on the branch, is unmistakably suggestive, leading to their reputation as a powerful aphrodisiac. Young girls were forbidden to pick them. The flesh is luscious and has a sensuous texture.

Sweet basil is said to stimulate sex drive and instil a sense of wellbeing.

Radishes were valued as a divine aphrodisiac by the ancient Egyptians, perhaps because their peppery flavour tickled the palate, or perhaps because of their colour and shape.

Fennel is regarded as a sexual stimulant in India, as it was by the ancient Greeks.

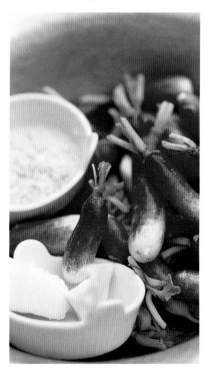

◄ Dipping radishes in soft butter and then salt is a traditional French hors d'oeuvres.

22 asparagus to share

There's no denying the phallic connotations of asparagus. For a delicious, sensuous experience, feed your lover the tender spears, with melted butter or the unctuous dressing in this recipe.

It's said that you should eat asparagus for three days for the most powerful effect – why not try it during its brief in-season period, when there is plenty of it about?

asparagus with creamy raspberry vinaigrette
350g/³⁄₄lb asparagus spears
15ml/1 tbsp raspberry vinegar
2.5ml/½ tsp Dijon mustard
45ml/3 tbsp sunflower oil
15ml/1 tsp soured cream
salt and white pepper
a few fresh raspberries

1 Fill a wide pan with water and bring to the boil. Trim the ends of the asparagus spears. Lower into the water and cook for 2 minutes or until just tender. Remove with a slotted spoon and drain. Leave to cool while you make the dressing.

2 Blend the vinegar with the mustard then gradually stir in the oil. Add the soured cream and season to taste.

3 Drizzle the dressing over the asparagus and serve with raspberries.

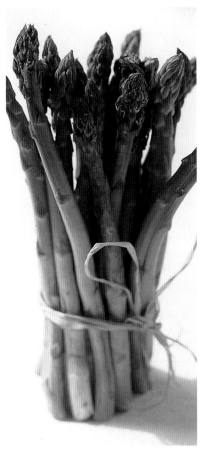

▲ Use the young slender spears for the tenderest taste experience.

23 luxurious seafood

A seafood feast is a fantastic start to a night of hedonistic pleasure. Choose lobster for sheer indulgence, or go for the classic seductive combination of oysters and champagne.

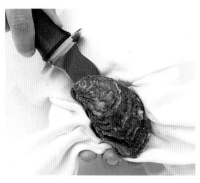

▲ Opening oysters and feeding them to your partner can make an entire love feast.

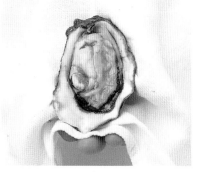

▲ Oysters not only feel sensuous, but they have an undeniably sexy appearance.

Fish of all kinds rightly claim a place on the list of aphrodisiacs – Aphrodite did, after all, emerge from the sea. They're also very nutritious, high in protein to keep up your stamina, zinc to increase testosterone levels, and Omega-3 fatty acids for circulation.

Apart from being a luxurious treat, oysters are the ultimate in sensual eating. Soft and wet, they slip smoothly down the throat, and their little folds and fissures give them an unmistakable resemblance to female genitalia. Made for feeding to each other: an oyster feast is the perfect party for two.

buying and preparing oysters
Make sure the shells are firmly shut when you buy oysters. Scrub the shells and keep them flat-side up to retain all the juices. Keep them cool, and eat them on the same day.

To open an oyster, grasp it firmly in a cloth with the hinge towards you. Press the point of the oyster knife into the hinge and rotate it to dislodge the upper shell. Slide the blade over the meat to sever the upper muscle. Do the same under the meat to free the oyster. Remove any fragments of shell and eat with lemon juice, black pepper and a drop of Tabasco.

24 turning up the heat

Spicy foods are viewed as aphrodisiacs because their effects on the body – raising the heart rate and making you sweat – are similar to some of the reactions experienced during sex.

Curry is full of tantalizing flavours and is great food to share.

Thai green chicken curry

450ml/¾ pint/2 cups chicken stock
2 boneless, skinless chicken breasts
200ml/7fl oz can coconut milk
30ml/2 tbsp chopped fresh coriander (cilantro)
shredded spring onions (scallions) and shredded red (bell) pepper, to serve

For the green curry paste:

5 fresh green chillies, chopped
6 shallots, chopped
3 garlic cloves
75g/3oz fresh coriander (cilantro)
finely grated rind of 1 lime
5ml/1 tsp dried shrimp paste
small piece of fresh root ginger, chopped
1 small stick lemon grass, chopped
2.5ml/½ tsp ground turmeric
2.5ml/½ tsp ground cumin
10ml/2 tsp ground coriander
30ml/2 tbsp vegetable oil
salt and ground black pepper

1 Make the green curry paste by processing all the ingredients until smooth. Whisk a little of the stock with about half the curry paste in a frying pan (the rest will keep, refrigerated, for about a month). Bring to the boil and simmer for about 2 minutes until the liquid has evaporated. Slice the chicken into strips.

3 Add the chicken and remaining stock and stir. Bring to the boil and simmer for 10 minutes. Stir in the coconut milk and simmer for 5 minutes.

4 Add the coriander and season to taste. Serve sprinkled with shredded spring onions and red pepper.

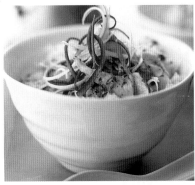

▲ Whether or not chillies really do lift your libido, this is a wonderfully warming dish.

25 nuts and honey

Drizzle honey over Greek yogurt and scatter it liberally with nuts and you'll be benefiting from two ancient sex secrets of the Mediterranean. It'll also make a delicious start to breakfast in bed.

For centuries, nuts have been mixed with honey for love potions. The Arabic sex manual, *The Perfumed Garden,* recommends a glass of thick honey, twenty almonds and a hundred pine nuts, repeated for three nights, to restore a man's sexual vigour.

Pine nuts are widely regarded as an aphrodisiac, and they are in fact a good source of zinc, which is said to boost the sex drive by raising

RUNNY HONEY
Drizzle a trail over your partner's body that you can then lick off – or plot a path over yourself and lead your lover in any direction you want.

testosterone levels. So serve lashings of fresh pesto with pasta, or toast the nuts and scatter them over salads.

The smell of almonds is supposed to induce passion in women, and they have long been a symbol of fertility, as are walnuts (which the Romans threw at newlyweds). All kinds of nuts are good energy foods.

honey
The Egyptians used honey as a cure for most things, including impotence. The honeymoon gets its name from the time when couples were encouraged to drink mead – made from fermented honey – to keep them going. Honey is high in B vitamins and amino acids which keep the body performing at its peak.

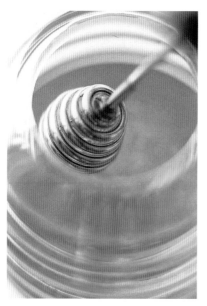

◄ *Honey has been given all kinds of medical and mystical properties through the ages.*

26 irresistible chocolate

Any erotic feast has to include a liberal supply of chocolate. It's said that chocolate contains a natural substance that causes the same physical reaction as falling in love.

Casanova described hot chocolate as "the elixir of love" and drank it instead of champagne. Chocolate's reputation for stimulating sexual desire came to Europe with the Spanish conquistadors, and whether or not it's true, the idea has been firmly fixed ever since. Modern adverts, particularly those aimed at women, are heavy with innuendo associating chocolate with indulgent passion. Dark chocolate, particularly, is clearly associated with wicked pleasures.

One of the reasons we love chocolate so much is the pure physical pleasure we get from the whole experience of eating it: not just its taste, but its heavy perfume and smooth, melting texture. The flavour of chocolate – two and a half times more complex than any other food – overwhelms the tastebuds, just as good sex overwhelms the body.

So chocolate's X-rated character makes it a winner in love-making. Simply melted by itself, or turned into a velvety mousse or a glistening sauce, it will trail beguilingly over warm skin, wherever you'd most enjoy having it licked off.

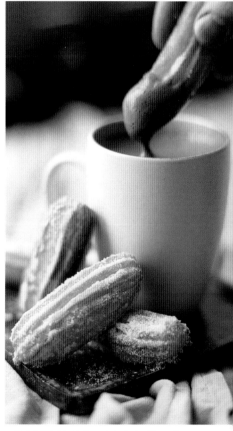

▲ Drink thick hot chocolate in bed together, morning or night, and dip crisp, warm churros into it for a powerful energy surge .

Choose **perfect cherries**, strawberries or seedless grapes and dip them in melted white chocolate. When that's set, dip them again in dark bitter chocolate and chill.

Take them to bed with you and feed them to each other.

28 fruity passion

Tropical fruit has it all: redolent of steamy jungle climates (even if it actually grew in a glasshouse), it tastes, smells, looks and feels sexy. What you do with it is limited only by your imagination.

We can buy exotic fruits every day of the year. Though this has robbed them of their rarity value, the allure of forbidden fruit still clings to them. When you pull open a fig its glowing red interior and soft, juicy flesh can't help but remind you, as it did D.H. Lawrence, of "The wonderful moist conductivity towards the centre" of a woman. Ripe papayas and guavas also conceal seed-filled, scented interiors of luminous colour. Mangoes should be eaten only in the bath. It's impossible to sink your teeth into the flesh of a mango without the juice running down your chin and arms, so it seems only sensible to take off all your clothes first.

Mix an exotic fruit cocktail with clementines, fresh figs, orange sorbet (sherbet), and spiced port, as an ideal midnight snack, or a light finish to a rich meal. Just pile the fruit and sorbet into glasses, warm the port with brown sugar, cinnamon and honey, until the sugar and honey have melted, and then pour it on the fruit.

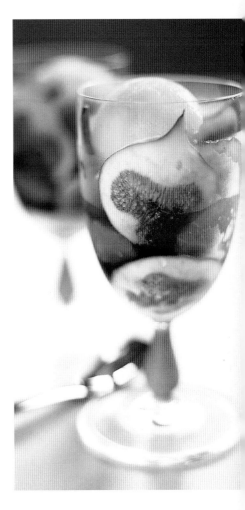

▸ *An exotic sundae can be made with any mixture of delicious fruits.*

29

popping corks

A little alcohol lowers inhibitions and increases confidence. Tease your senses with iced champagne or a voluptuous cocktail. But beware the dangers of drinking too much.

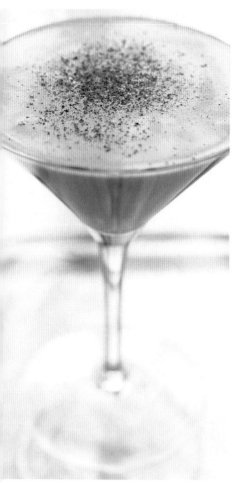

A couple of glasses of wine definitely help to create the right mood for an enjoyable romp, and could give you or your partner the confidence to try something daring and new.

Drinking wine is relaxing but it also stimulates all the senses, as you smell its complex aroma and savour its taste. As for champagne, who wouldn't feel sexier when its gentle little bubbles are tickling the nose? It envelops you in a warm, rosy glow and adds a note of celebration to the encounter – which is always flattering and romantic.

Casanova cocktail
1 measure/1 ½ tbsp bourbon
½ measure/2 tsp marsala dolce
½ measure/2 tsp Kahlua
1 measure/1 ½ tbsp double
    (heavy) cream

Shake all the ingredients well with plenty of ice to amalgamate the cream. Strain into a glass. Sprinkle with ground nutmeg.

◀ *This creamy cocktail looks almost as good as it tastes.*

30 aromatherapy bath oils

Turn your bathroom into a sensual haven with a gorgeously indulgent scented bath. Essential oils will get you in the mood for passion, and their scent will linger enticingly on your skin.

Just sprinkle 4-6 drops of your favourite essential oil on the surface of the water after you have drawn the bath and agitate the water to mix it. Don't add essential oils while the water is running, because much of the fragrant vapour will have dispersed before you get into the bath. If you want to soothe and moisturize dry skin, you can mix the essential oils with a carrier oil such as sweet almond, and add some wheatgerm oil which is high in skin-nourishing vitamin E.

Rose and sandalwood bath oil
A little rose essential oil goes a long way, as it has a powerful fragrance. When combined with sandalwood it creates a warm, spicy fragrance.

100ml/3 ½ fl oz almond oil
20ml/4 tsp wheatgerm oil
15 drops rose essential oil
10 drops sandalwood essential oil

Pour the almond and wheatgerm oils into a bottle, add the essential oils and shake. Add a tablespoon to the bath.

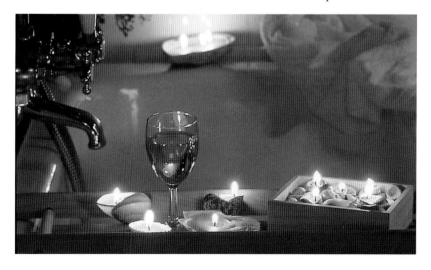

31

smooth silky skin

Toning scrubs for the face and body are great for gently exfoliating and stimulating the blood supply to the skin. They'll leave you tingling and revitalized.

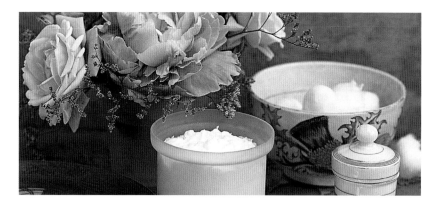

Citrus body scrub

Makes enough for 5 treatments
45ml/3 tbsp freshly ground sunflower
    seeds
45ml/3 tbsp medium oatmeal
45ml/3 tbsp flaked sea salt
45ml/3 tbsp finely grated orange peel
3 drops grapefruit essential oil
almond oil

Mix all the ingredients except the almond oil and store in a sealed jar. To use, mix to a paste with almond oil and rub over the body, paying particular attention to areas of hard skin such as the elbows and knees, then shower off.

▲ *Use roses to scent your bathroom as well as in your facial scrub.*

Gentle facial scrub

Makes enough for 10 treatments
30ml/2 tbsp dried rose petals
45ml/3 tbsp ground almonds
45ml/3 tbsp medium oatmeal
45ml/3 tbsp powdered milk
almond oil

Powder the rose petals in a pestle and mortar or electric grinder. Mix all the dry ingredients and store in a sealed jar. Mix to a paste with almond oil. Rub into the face, avoiding the eyes, and rinse off with warm water.

Prolong the intimacy of touch by sharing a long, indulgent bath filled with fragrant bubbles, and revel in the silky warmth caressing your skin.

33 delicious dusting powder

Don't think of talcum powder as the province of babies and old ladies. A light dusting over clean warm skin makes it feel satiny and is a wonderful way to coat the body with gentle fragrance.

You can make your own dusting powder from scratch, or use unscented talc as a base. Either way, you'll create a luxurious scented powder that's a world away from commercial brands. Pat it all over with a huge swansdown puff to make yourself feel like a star.

Luscious lavender body powder
60ml/4 tbsp white kaolin clay
60ml/4 tbsp arrowroot
75ml/5 tbsp cornflour
3 drops each lavender, coriander,
   lemon and geranium essential oils

Mix the kaolin, arrowroot and 60ml/4 tbsp of the cornflour. Add the essential oils to the remaining cornflour and stir into the powder.

single fragrance dusting powder
This is simple to make with ready-made unscented talc. To every 5 tablespoons of talc add 1 tablespoon of cornflour, scented with 5 drops of essential oil. Try jasmine or ylang ylang for a heavy, seductive scent, or rose for a more romantic effect.

▾ *Apply your talc with a luxurious powder puff to give an extra glamorous feel.*

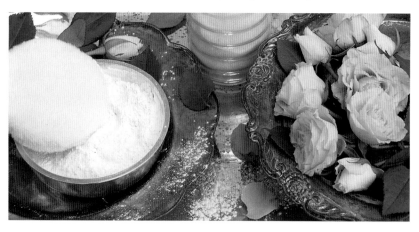

34 shimmering tresses

Historically, no part of a woman's body has aroused more adulation than her hair. Throughout the ages, flowing locks have been praised in poetry and celebrated in art.

The fifth-century Sanskrit poet Bhartrhari described a woman's hair as a forest, enticing the explorer into unknown territory where love waits like a bandit to ambush him. Luxuriant hair exerts a powerful sexual allure. In some cultures, it is still kept hidden to avoid tempting men.

Apart from hairdressers and masseurs, few people actually touch our heads, so running the fingers through a lover's hair is an intimate gesture. The scent of hair is personal and potent – perfume lingers longer in the hair than anywhere else, so a spritz of fragrance makes it irresistible.

Rinses made from herbs rather than chemicals give a much fresher, natural scent and will also nourish the hair.

herbal hair rinse

A simple herbal rinse gives your hair a wonderful fresh fragrance and leaves it smooth and lustrous. Pour a cup of boiling water over a handful of fresh lemon verbena leaves, or fresh parsley, and leave to infuse for at least an hour. Strain the liquid, discarding the leaves, and use as a final rinse after washing.

▾ Herbs such as lemon verbena and parsley condition as well as scent your hair.

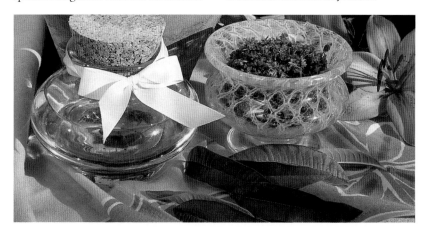

35

mint foot treatments

A foot massage can be a great turn-on. Feet are among the most sensitive areas of the body, and once you start to pamper them you may begin to see them as a seriously sexy zone.

Feet are too often tired, sore and rather neglected, but making them feel good can revitalize your whole body. Mint is a refreshing cooler for hot, aching feet and leaves them smelling sweet and feeling soothed.

Mint footbath
12 large sprigs mint
120ml/4fl oz/½ cup cold water
2.4 litres/4 pints/10 cups hot water

Place the mint in a food processor with the cold water and blend to a

green purée. Add to the boiling water in a large bowl and leave to cool to a bearable temperature before soaking the feet.

Mint massage oil
15ml/1 tbsp almond oil
1 drop mint essential oil

Mix the oils and rub well into the feet, then begin the massage.

▼ A massage may begin as a therapeutic exercise but lead to other things.

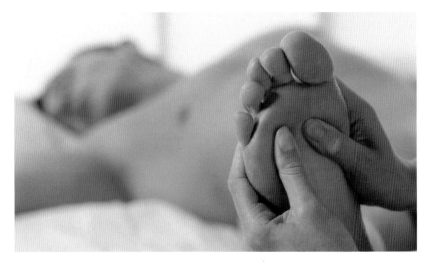

36 colour magic

People have a powerful response to colour. If you want your bedroom to feel vibrant, stimulating and just a little bit dangerous, add some cushions or throws in vibrant red.

It's impossible to be indifferent to colour. It surrounds us all the time. Its influence on mood is obvious: just imagine walking between concrete walls, sitting in the shade of a leafy tree, gazing into a clear blue sky, or putting on a bright red sweater, and you can immediately appreciate the power of colour.

feeling red

Red is the nearest visible light to heat in the electromagnetic spectrum. We connect it with heat and the danger of burning. It's the colour of smouldering coals, and lava erupting from a volcano. As the colour of blood red has links with life and liveliness. It signifies activity, daring and passion.

Phrases like "red light district" and "scarlet woman" bring out the sexual nature of red – not just sexy, but illicit – naughty rather than nice. It's an immediate colour, restless and impatient. It's associated with the expression of emotions – whether passion, anger or aggression – that can be hard to handle and make the heart beat faster, the capillaries dilate and the skin flushed and warm.

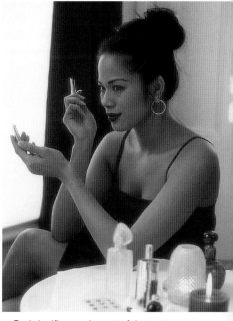

▲ Red signifies an element of danger to others, and gives you a feeling of daring.

So a red bedroom might not give you peaceful sleep, but if you want to generate vitality, boldness and passion, it's the colour to choose. Rather than painting the room red though, you could always use moveable items such as drapes and cushions.

37 setting the scene

Your bedroom is one of the most important rooms in your home: make it a warm cocoon of comfort and an intimate space for lovemaking and sensuality.

We spend more time in the bedroom than in any other single room, so creating the right atmosphere here can have a profound effect on how we feel all the time. The room needs to be a sanctuary, where intimate exchanges can take place in a relaxed and harmonious way.

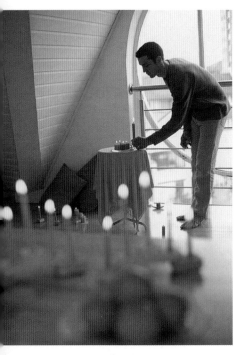

Anything connected with the outside world should be kept to a minimum and should be out of sight. That means clearing clutter. Put clothes and shoes away, and never allow anything to do with work to creep into the bedroom. A computer is definitely a bad idea, and apart from essential items, it's better if all electrical appliances are kept somewhere else.

softness and warmth
The bed – the larger the better – clearly needs to take centre stage, without too many other pieces of furniture competing for attention. Hang billowing silk drapes or netting around the bed for a romantic, theatrical effect. A rich, sensuous haven will set the scene for intimacy, with soft, luxurious textures complemented by warm low-level lighting. Deep, warm pinks and reds are perfect, but don't use colours that are so strong and bright that you can't eventually fall into restful sleep.

◀ *Set the scene for a night of love throughout the house, not just the bedroom.*

Make your bed a dream of comfort, with a cloud-soft duvet, the smoothest, coolest sheets and a mountain of pillows.

39 romantic lighting

The right lighting can create a magical space, whether you're preparing the bathroom for an evening of sensual solitude or setting the scene for seduction in the bedroom.

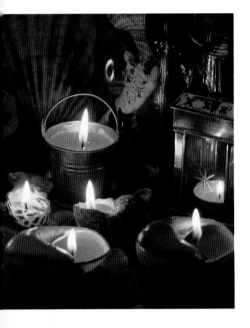

◀ *Candlelight can't be beaten for creating a beautiful glow, and a relaxing atmosphere.*

Fairylights or christmas lights also cast a gentle but exciting light and are very flattering. String them around the bedhead to lend enchantment and magic to the proceedings.

seashell candles
You can scent these enchanting little candles by adding a seductive essential oil to the wax.
clean shells
sand-filled bowl
150g/5oz paraffin wax
50g/2oz natural beeswax
double boiler
metal-core wick for small candles
waxed paper

1 Steady the shells in the sand-filled bowl. Melt the waxes together in a double boiler. Prime the wicks by soaking the lengths in the wax and leave to cool on waxed paper.

2 Pour the hot wax into the shells (do not overfill). Leave until partially set then push in the primed wicks.

The warm glow of candlelight is the most flattering of all, smoothing away imperfections and giving skin a luminous sheen. Flickering candle flames have a hypnotic, relaxing effect. Create an extravagant, fantastic scene by filling the room with candles, or light just a few near the bed for an intimate, cavelike effect in an otherwise darkened room.

40 scents for seduction

The sense of smell is the most primitive of our five senses, and perfumes of all kinds are powerful triggers of both physical and emotional responses. Scent and sex are inextricably linked.

Legend has it that Mark Antony had to wade through a carpet of rose petals in order to reach Cleopatra's bed, and perfume is a traditional gift of love. But the scent most strongly redolent of sex is the natural smell of bodies.

erogenic scents

Like plants and animals, a natural aroma is part of our biological strategy for attracting a mate. Hormone-like chemicals, known as pheromones, are scent signals radiated by the skin. Certain animal and plant fragrances resemble human pheromones, and can be used to stimulate sexual desire. They are known as erogenic aromas.

Musk, a secretion of the musk deer, is probably the most famous, with its earthy, sensuous scent. Erogenic aromas are also found in jasmine, rose, ylang ylang and patchouli.

using scent

The bedroom can be subtly scented with fragrant oils, scented candles or flowers. Scatter rose petals on the bed, scent linen when you wash and iron it, and spray perfume in a fine mist over the carpet so that the fragrance is released when you walk on it.

▾ *Scent your bedroom with fresh flower heads and bowls of essential oils.*

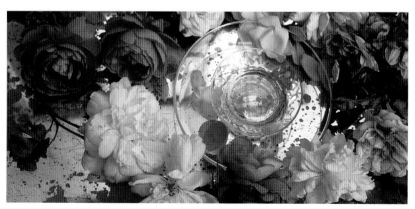

41

sexy essential oils

Essential oils can be used in many ways to cast their spell on your senses. They are concentrated substances, each with its own characteristics and properties, and their effects can be profound.

The erotic charge of these aromas has made them famous as ingredients of love potions and perfume blends designed for seduction. Use them in aromatherapy burners, in oil blends for massage or to fragrance baths.

jasmine
The warm, exotic smell of jasmine has a musky undertone, and has been used for centuries in love potions and bridal garlands. Its euphoric effect can liberate sexual fantasies.

ylang ylang
The relaxing effect of this intensely sweet scent reduces stress levels and removes inhibition.

neroli
Orange blossom is reputed to raise the libido, lull inhibitions and allow secret desires to be expressed.

clary sage
This heady, sweet aroma has a euphoric and relaxing effect.

▸ *Establish an aromatherapy burner in your room and a selection of essential oils.*

sandalwood
Probably the oldest perfume in history, sandalwood's heavy scent can lift depression that often causes sexual problems.

rose
The rose is a symbol of love and romantic longing. Its wonderful fragrance evokes general feelings of pleasure and happiness.

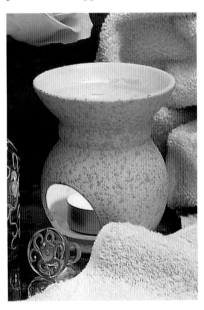

42 pillow talk

Talking about your innermost feelings can be difficult, but one of the most successful ways to keep a relationship flourishing is by being best friends and being open with each other.

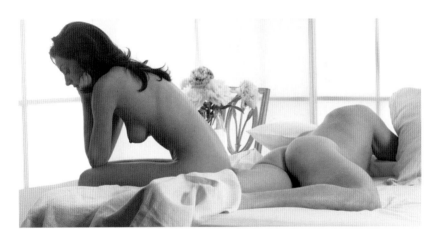

It takes time to build up trust and feel able to talk about your fantasies, fears and needs, but communication is key in every relationship. It's important to let the other person know what you are feeling or expecting, not just to avoid misunderstandings but to get what you want.

Are there things you'd love your partner to try? Is there something a little perverse that you'd like to do during sex but are too embarrassed to suggest? Is there anything you don't really like your partner doing, but don't want to mention?

▲ Communication is vital for a healthy relationship and an active sex life.

sexual communication

Direct criticism can be upsetting and intimidating. The best way to tell your partner about your likes and dislikes is by affirmation: "I love it when you touch me there," for example, or "It feels better this way." Once you've opened a channel of communication in this positive way, it may be easier to talk about things that are a problem for you, and to open the way for your partner to do the same.

43 loving face massage

Slowly, gently massaging your lover's face with awareness and sensitivity can be a very intimate, sensual experience for both of you. Enhance the massage by using some essential oils.

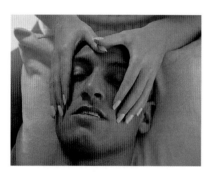

1 Apply a small quantity of oil to your hands. Use them to stroke gently, one after the other, first up over the neck, and then across the chin and jaw, up to the forehead. Glide your thumbs steadily from the centre of the brow towards the sides of the head. Repeat the stroke up over the entire forehead. Rotate your fingertips anti-clockwise on one place all over the cheeks.

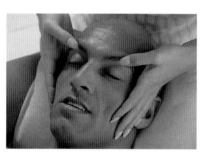

2 Draw your thumbs from the inner to the outer edges of the eyebrows, then press the pads sensitively up into and along the brow bone. Repeat the movement down the nose, beginning at the bridge and moving your thumbs down to the nostrils then out towards the cheekbones.

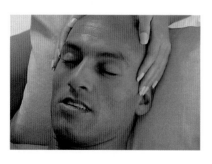

3 Relax your hands to sweep the palms soothingly up over the sides of the temples and scalp, then draw them away from the head. Softly cup your hands, circling your fingertips several times in soothing clockwise motions over your partner's temples. Complete the massage by cradling the head between your hands.

44 sensual touch

The most important element of sensual massage is the caring presence of your hands on your partner's body. Allow your intuition to show you how and where to apply the strokes.

After a stressful day, massaging your partner allows you time to wind down and get back in touch with one another. It need not be a precursor to sex, but it can set the scene and get you both in the mood.

Pour a little oil into your hands and warm them by rubbing them together before you begin. Long, sweeping strokes over the back can be performed while straddling your partner's hips. This keeps you in close contact, but you should support your own weight. Maintain a constant, confident touch, using long, flowing unbroken strokes. Your hands should encompass fully the contours of the body, such as the shoulders, hips and buttocks.

▼ *Your touch can be at times soft, gentle and nurturing or firm and stimulating.*

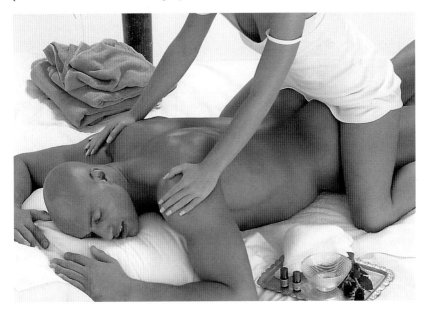

kissing asides

There's a whole repertoire of kissing to try out: not all kisses have to involve tickling each other's tonsils. In the right circumstances an almost imperceptible brush of the lips can be just as exciting.

Women tend to like kissing better than men, and enjoy the whole, long, lingering embrace, without it necessarily leading on to anything else. Some women say that they find kissing the most erotic part of sex, whereas men tend to see it as a step on the way to intercourse. What makes a great kiss? Here are a few suggestions:

french kissing: Gently caress the inside of your partner's mouth with your tongue. As they respond, you can quicken the pace and intensity, going for a fuller thrust.

chicken kisses: Great for moments of tenderness. Plant light pecks at the rate of about three a second. It's between a kiss and a tickle, but feels good.

stereophonic kiss: Some people adore the sound and sensation of being kissed inside their ears – the slooshing sound really turns them on.

talking kiss: Hold your partner's face between your hands and kiss different parts of it – each eyebrow, each eyelid, nose, cheeks – and between each kiss say something erotic: what you're about to do to them, what you'd like them to do to you, and so on.

butterfly kiss: Use your eyelashes to brush against your partner's face or body.

love bites: Think twice before you bite, they hurt.

◀ *Kissing sometimes gets abandoned in a long established relationship. Try and revive it if that is the case in yours.*

Play with an ice cube: try sliding it over your bodies, passing it from mouth to mouth. The sensation of iced water against hot skin excites nerve endings in a way that hands and fingers can't.

47 sexplorations

For a truly sensual experience, take a journey around your partner's body. Think of it as a luscious and varied landscape: instead of the familiar places, visit the parts you've hardly explored.

How often has your partner absently stroked the inside of your wrist, sending electrifying spasms through your body? Sometimes the less obvious parts of the body create the biggest thrills. Focusing on different areas shows that you find your partner sexy all over, not just at the hotspots.

erogenous zones
The back of the neck is a very relaxing and loving place to caress a lover, as it has a mysterious link to the body's sensual centres. It sends a mixture of warm and thrilling shock waves along the entire length of the spine, leaving you feeling energized and loved.

The navel is another extremely sensitive area. Some people are a bit squeamish about it, but others love having their belly buttons caressed by a soft tongue.

Fingers are an understandably popular focus of attention, because their tips are so sensitive, and sucking the fingers is loaded with innuendo. The toes are just as sensitive, but sucking them is something that people either love or hate. Some find it a real turn-on. For those who can

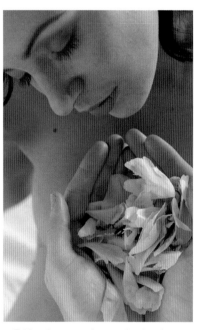

▲ Taking time to explore each others' bodies will help your love making.

bear to have their feet touched, the instep is another nerve-rich area. Many people love to have their feet massaged and pampered. Using your toes can also be an interesting way to stimulate other areas of your partner's body (as long as your feet aren't cold).

48 playing games

Sex isn't something that needs to be taken seriously, it should be fun. If things are becoming repetitive in your relationship, it's time to spice up your love-making with some fun and games.

There are lots of possibilities: you can play strip poker, naked Scrabble, or hide and seek. Why not adapt the rules of the games and introduce some forfeits of your own?

dice game

Get two dice. Write down a sexual position for each number on the first die. Then write down six locations for the second. Roll the dice together and obey dutifully.

▾ *Ring your partner on his mobile from the bedroom and indulge in some sex talk.*

sex with a stranger

Here's an idea for an anniversary surprise. Invite your partner to meet you for a meal, both pretending you are strangers on a blind date.

Spend the evening flirting as you did when you first met. At the end of the evening suggest a one-night stand in the hotel room nearby (that you've already secretly booked). If you can stay in character, playing the consummate sexual host or hostess and doing anything your partner requests, this should guarantee some passionate and exciting sex.

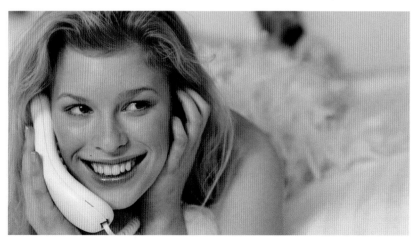

49 erotica

Reading erotic literature stimulates the erogenous zone that full-on pornography simply can't reach – the brain. Read it alone, or together, or to each other, for a great turn-on.

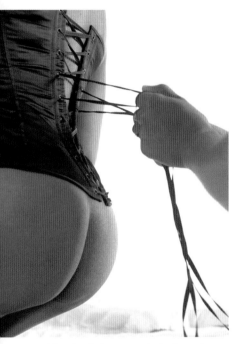

◄ *The simplest prop can instantly conjure up a storm of sexual meaning.*

Erotic literature and films can be a great aid to sex, whether you use them as a warm-up act beforehand or read them together in bed. The choice of novels, poetry and magazines is huge these days. They can provide you with ready-made scenarios to act out between you, or inspire and embellish your own fantasies.

Your favourite sensual or erotic films are guaranteed to get you in the mood: you might be inspired by a raunchy modern sex scene or by the buttoned-up restraint of a costume drama, where desire has to smoulder under the surface.

pornography
At the other end of the scale, gritty porn films and dirty magazines can be exciting because of their complete lack of subtlety. They can help you express desires and fantasies that you would probably never act upon. They might even give you some interesting ideas, or they might just make you roar with laughter together.

If you have a camcorder you could try making your own porn film. Choose your roles and dress up appropriately, position the camera with a good view of the bed and off you go. Watching it afterwards can be extremely erotic – seeing yourselves making love from a different angle gives you a whole new perspective.

50 sharing fantasies

People guard their fantasies fiercely, regardless of how close they are to their partner. It can be liberating to share some of yours with your lover, and even more so to act them out.

Humans have very complex brains, and it's often not enough just to stimulate the genitals to feel sexually fulfilled. We have to be in just the correct mood before we are relaxed enough to let our bodies go, and our personal fantasies can provide the right mind-set.

Some fantasies are simple enough to enact: having sex in an exclusive and elegant hotel, being wooed in a romantic candlelit room, or being swept away by passion on a warm and sunny cliff-top. Others that involve a cast of thousands, all acting in the way your fantasy requires, aren't so easy.

Having sex with a celebrity is a common fantasy. If you try this one while having sex with your partner it won't do any harm – as long as you don't scream out the wrong name at the wrong time.

private thoughts

Many people are embarassed by the content of their fantasies, and worry that they imagine weird or illegal acts, but it's worth remembering that it's human instinct to be drawn precisely to whatever's forbidden.

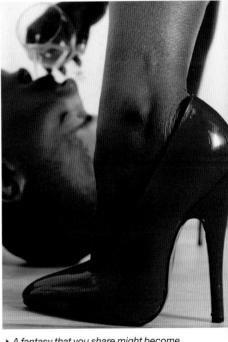

▸ A fantasy that you share might become an enjoyable part of your sex life.

Keep your fantasies as a private store of erotic movies that you can switch on whenever you like. Your brain is the biggest and most powerful sex organ you have and where the mind leads, the body will follow.

index

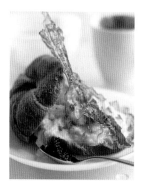

affirmations 20
agnus castus 25
alcohol 7, 40
alpha state 19
aphrodisiacs 10, 31
appearance 15
aromatherapy bath oils 41
asparagus 33

bathing 41, 43
bedrooms 48-9
borage 26
breathing 23
buttercup 26

candles 8, 50
Casanova, 37
    Casanova cocktail 40
caviar 31
champagne 30, 34, 40
chocolate 8, 37, 38
citrus body scrub 42
Cleopatra 51
colour 47, 48
confidence 6, 15, 20

crystals 27

daffodil 26
damiana 24
dandelion 26
dating 12, 13
depression 6, 7
dice game 59
diet 6, 29, 32
drugs 6, 7
dusting powder 44

eating together 30
endorphins 16
erogenic scents 51
erogenous zones 58
erotica 60
essential oils 52
exercise 6, 16-18
    yoga 22-3

face massage 54
fantasies 61
feet 28, 46
flower essences 26
fruit 38, 39

fugu (puffer fish) 31

games 59
gentle facial scrub 42
graphites 25

hair 45
health 6
herbs 24
    herbal hair rinse 45
homeopathy 25
honey 36
hormones 6, 16, 51

insomnia 21

jasmine 8, 10, 52

Kegel, Dr Arnold 18
kissing 56-7
Korean ginseng 24

lavender body powder 44
Lawrence, D. H. 39
lighting 8, 10, 50
lycopodium 25

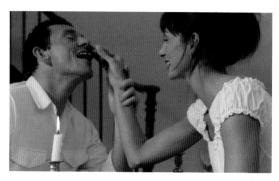

index

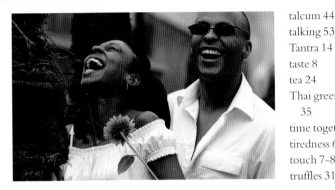

mangoes 8, 39
Mark Antony 51
massage 28, 46, 54, 55
meditation 19
midnight feasts 30
minerals 29
mint footbath and massage
    oil 46
music 8

natrum mur 25
nutrition 6, 29, 32
nuts 36

oysters 8, 10, 30, 34

pelvic floor muscles 18
Perfumed Garden, The 36
pillow talk 53
pornography 60
private thoughts 61
red 47
reflexology 28
rose and sandalwood bath
    oil 41

salads 32
scent 8, 10, 41, 44, 51, 52
scrubs 42
seafood 34
seashell candles 50
seduction 12, 51
self-esteem 6, 15, 20
sensuality 7
sepia 25
sex with a stranger game
    59
sexplorations 58
sight 8
single fragrance dusting
    powder 44
skin 42, 43
sleep 21
smoking 6-7
snake blood 31
softness 48
spicy foods 35
stress 6, 10, 21
    exercise 16, 17
stretches 17

talcum 44
talking 53
Tantra 14
taste 8
tea 24
Thai green chicken curry
    35
time together 14
tiredness 6, 10, 21
touch 7-8, 43, 55
truffles 31

vegetables 32, 33
vervain 24
vitamins 29

warmth 48
wild oats 24
wine 8, 40

yoga 22-3

zinnia 26

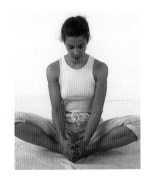

This edition is published by Lorenz Books

Lorenz Books is an imprint of Anness Publishing Ltd
Hermes House, 88–89 Blackfriars Road, London SE1 8HA
tel. 020 7401 2077; fax 020 7633 9499
www.lorenzbooks.com; info@anness.com

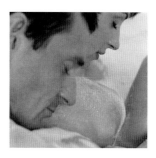

UK agent: The Manning Partnership Ltd,
6 The Old Dairy,
Melcombe Road, Bath BA2 3LR;
tel. 01225 478 444; fax 01225 478 440;
sales@manning-partnership.co.uk

UK distributor: Grantham Book Services
Ltd, Isaac Newton Way,
Alma Park Industrial Estate, Grantham,
Lincs NG31 9SD;
tel. 01476 541 080; fax 01476 541 061;
orders@gbs.tbs-ltd.co.uk

North American agent/distributor:
National Book Network,
4501 Forbes Boulevard, Suite 200,
Lanham, MD 20706;
tel. 301 459 3366; fax 301 429 5746;
www.nbnbooks.com

Australian agent/distributor:
Pan Macmillan Australia, Level 18,
St Martins Tower, 31 Market St,
Sydney, NSW 2000;
tel. 1300 135 113; fax 1300 135 103;
customer.service@macmillan.com.au

New Zealand agent/distributor:
David Bateman Ltd,
30 Tarndale Grove, Off Bush Road,
Albany, Auckland;
tel. (09) 415 7664; fax (09) 415 8892

A CIP catalogue record for this book is
available from the British Library.

Publisher: Joanna Lorenz
Editorial Director: Helen Sudell
Executive Editor: Joanne Rippin
Designer: Adelle Morris
Production controller: Darren Price

10 9 8 7 6 5 4 3 2 1

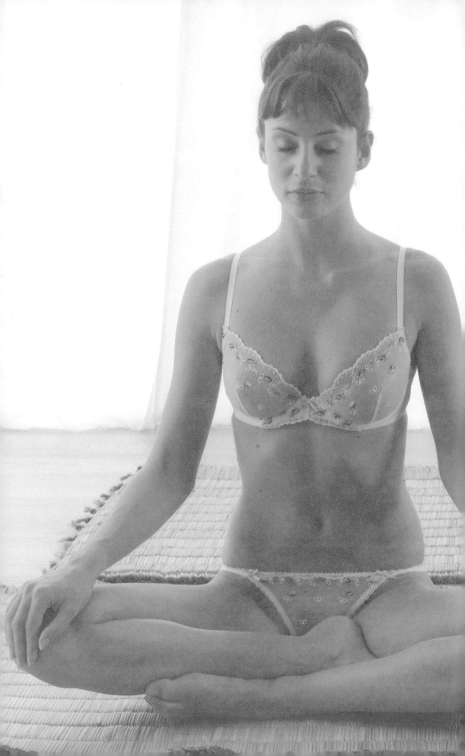